THE PUBLIC FORUMS ON THE EBOLA VACCINE TRIALS IN GHANA

FOUR REPORTS FROM FREELANCE REPORTERS

I0401455

AUTHORS

Isaac Ato Mensah

Ahmed Naeem Abdul-Ghafaar

Ekow Arthur-Aidoo

Emmanuel Amoh Kwaning

Stella Owusu Kwarteng

Published by

writersghana.com

Cover photograph

The Atewa Range Forest Reserve, 2019

DEDICATION

To the victims of Ebola

ACKNOWLEDGEMENTS

We are grateful to Mr Tony Goodman for the connection and facilitating our transport.

ABOUT THE BOOK

There were four Public Forums organised in Ghana in 2015 to engage the general public about the Ebola epidemic in West Africa. We, the authors, connected informally with Tony Goodman, the Public Relations Officer (PRO) of the Ministry of Health at the time and he facilitated our trips to the various venues. We gave him same-day reports as independent reporters. We are proud of our contribution since it helped to relax the nerves of the officials of the Ministry of Health as well as Members of Parliament, thereby ensuring progress on the basis of facts, evidence and reason. The confusion about whether or not there was an Ebola vaccine in Ghana was caused by reporters/journalists. And it took us - freelance reporters - to dispel those rumours by listening to all the facts, preparing same day reports and drawing firm conclusions for the PRO. The palpable tension was such that credibility in what the employed health experts/scientists were saying was at an all time low. Due to the tensions, we tried as much as possible to maintain some near verbatim comments and little to no editing of some contributions, while also boldly stating our understanding of the matter in our executive summaries. All the contents in this book is our compilation hence we take full responsibility for any errors.

TABLE OF CONTENTS

PART ONE

A REPORT OF THE OPEN FORUM ON THE EBOLA VACCINE TRIAL ORGANISED UNDER THE AUSPICES OF THE MINISTER OF HEALTH AT THE CIVIL SERVANTS AUDITORIUM, MINISTRIES, ACCRA ON THURSDAY 18TH JUNE, 2015

EXECUTIVE SUMMARY

There was breaking news recently about a supposedly sudden trial of Ebola vaccines in Ghana. There have been a lot of media responses and public reactions. The Honourable Minister of Health promised the parliament of Ghana to sponsor a public forum on the trial. The first forum was held at the Civil Servants Auditorium, Ministries, Accra.

The forum was well attended; the auditorium was almost full. Journalists and members of the general public attended. Very prominent health workers from the relevant agencies were invited to the high table to answer questions.

The speakers were very good at delivering their messages to the audience. Most of the audience agreed with them. Only a few issues remained not well communicated. One is the source of the alleged US$2800.00 to be given to study participants as opposed to the 200 Ghanaian cedis being offered. Nobody seemed to know the source of that US$2800.00 figure, yet it lingers. The second is why Ghana was chosen as a vaccine trial country. The answers given were very good. The answers should be played as sound bites on radio: Vaccine trials are undertaken in a healthy population. Ghana has the qualified scientists and regulatory expertise to manage vaccine trials.

One potent comment from the WHO Country Director resonated with participants: I know that in your hearts you all want a vaccine to be approved and you want to be the first to receive the vaccine in case of an outbreak. A second was also potent; Dr Antwi Adjei, a former director of the MOH/GHS said we have been doing trials for a long time just that we don't make *dedey* [noise] about it. This also got the audience laughing. A third was equally potent; the principal investigator from Kintampo said he is doing trials and paying GHC20.00 to participants. Now how can he explain to his study participants that some other persons are giving GHC200.00 and he is paying only GHC20.00? A fourth still potent response from the speakers is that if there is an Ebola outbreak, the MOH shall have the data to make a decision to use the experimental vaccines for its frontline staff because it has been tried in a healthy population in Ghana.

The Ghana Academy of Arts and Sciences received a bashing from the public for their absence. The essence of public relations is to meet each half way on a two-way symmetrical street. A special meeting should therefore be held with the Ghana Academy of Arts and Sciences with the media present. They should be allowed to bring up issues in a cordial manner.

Prof Binka (Hohoe) and Dr Kwaku Poku Asante (Kintampo) should be hosted on Adult Education on GTV, on Peace FM and other speaking platforms; they are very good communicators and they can think on their feet.

INTRODUCTION

Tony Goodman welcomed guests at 2:30PM and invited special guests to take their seats at the high table.

The Greater Accra Regional Health Director and a rep of the Food and Drugs Authority were invited to the high table. He then asked someone to say an opening prayer. After the opening prayer, the Principal Investigator at the Kintampo Health Research Centre was invited to join the high table.

He said that as the audience was aware, the Minister of Health had made it clear to the public and Members of Parliament that he would be conveying a stakeholders' forum on the Ebola Vaccine Phase One trial which is to commence in the Volta Region.

The Greater Accra Regional Health Director was invited to accept the chairperson's position for the function.

WELCOME ADDRESS

"It is an honour for me to be part of this discussion. We have questions on our mind; I stand here to welcome all of us," she said. "I hope all our confusion will be addressed by the end of the discussion. She said if someone is not satisfied, he/she should ask questions until he/she is satisfied. She thanked the media and thanked the organizers for asking her to chair the programme.

TONY GOODMAN

Mr Goodman said many people make comments on social media therefore there is a challenge to respond on social media as well. He then invited Prof Binka to speak.

PROF FRED BINKA, Chief investigator, University of Health and Allied Sciences

Why are we here?

I have been involved in vaccines for the past 25 years. I hope that as we begin this journey we will be able to help ourselves and do better next time.

Ghana was selected because it met the criteria required for vaccine trials.

This epidemic is not over. People remain at risk. It is important to protect all front line workers. New Ebola outbreaks will almost certainly be trembling. At this time there is no vaccine licensed for use in humans. Vaccines are taken through pre-clinical trial. Clinical trials have four phases.

Phase 1; Examine safety

Phase 2; Which vaccine is being tried?

Phase 3; Thousands of people are recruited as participants.

Phase 4; Post trial stage. At this stage any spontaneous reactions that occur are identified.

In Ghana, we are planning to start Phase 1.

Why was Hohoe Selected?

The World Health Organisation (WHO) has used Hohoe since 1986; the research centre is therefore highly recognized.

The Kintampo Health Centre has for the past decade been used for meningitis trials. The Centre has well equipped facilities for trial.

The USA, Switzerland, Germany, Mali and other countries are also getting participants in phase one of the vaccine trial.

The Chimpanzee Adenovirus is the main strain of virus being studied.

The process involves some viruses being knocked out and replaced with a protein. It sounds so simple but you need to know how to do it.

Vaccine trials have also taken place in Hohoe.

The Zaire strain which is being used in the Vaccine contains about 97 percent of the virus. The genes are knocked out and several proteins added.

The mapped virus known as Adenovirus and MVA undergo multiple gene deletions which render them replication incompetent. These two form the virus.

Who are the participants?

Healthy participants; You will have an exam to find out if you understand what you are about to undertake.

Your liver, spleen and every part of your body will be examined. In the case of women, pregnancy tests are mandatory. Pregnant women are not allowed to join. Once it is shown to be safe, later trials can involve pregnant women. Volunteers are not paid to take part in trials.

THE PROCESS OF CLINICAL TRIALS IN GHANA

Prof Binka explained that a trial centre has to express an interest and send an application form to the vaccine manufacturer. A questionnaire is sent to the institution. The site is selected and an inspection is done. The sponsor will then follow a protocol by informing the Food and Drug Authority of its intentions.

We then wait for approval from the FDA. We go through the trials and learn our lessons.

The final results will then be shared with participants. The study will be compared with other trial centres in the world. If approved by the regulatory authority, vaccines are given to countries that experience an outbreak. No individual who participated in the trial is identified.

DR KWAKU POKU ASANTE

I have been doing clinical trials in Kintampo since 2002. I have done trials for meningitis and malaria vaccines. My job here is to do a point by point comment on our response to the questions posed by our senior colleagues in the Ghana Academy of Arts and Sciences.

FIRST COMMENT

What are the strains of the Ebola virus?

There are different strains of the Ebola virus.

The question posed by the Ghana Academy of Arts and Science is about the nature of the strain of virus being used in this trial. The strain found in Zaire is what has been identified and is in the vaccine we want to test. The strain that runs in the epidemic around the world is about 97% of the strain we want to test.

Is the vaccine able to fight against different strains?

The strain in the vaccine is similar to the one that is in Guinea. At the moment we are not able to tell what other strain will come up. For many years we have been giving experimental vaccines that have two strains. The new outbreak had a different strain. Our own colleagues in Ghana did trials and found solutions.

Scientists will not sit on their oars and rest as outbreaks affect humans. Before any vaccine is given to humans, it is first tried in chimpanzees, who are closest to humans by scientific definition.

Do we have any data to show that the vaccine is safe in humans as per chimpanzee trials?

GSK has shown that the strain contains 97% of strains that have occurred in outbreaks.

Will there be an immune response to the vaccines being tried?

We have been checking to see if the vaccine is safe.

We are not doing an efficacy trial. If there is an outbreak, that will be the only time we will have to test if the medicine is efficacious or not. We are not bringing in sick people.

What is the assurance that vaccines do not carry a virus that will not cause disease in humans?

The days of using live viruses are almost gone. The part of the virus that has been taken away has to be carried on in another form. These are the germs that are being carried on.

How will it cause diseases?

It cannot.

The safety of our participants in clinical trials is very dear to us. Meanwhile other trials are being conducted in adults in the USA, the UK, Switzerland, Mali and other countries. It will not be given to children.

Always the first group of persons to receive a vaccine are healthy male adults. Women are excluded because we do not want babies affected.

The safety profile is decided by an independent group of scientists who have knowledge of scientific data and cultural settings.

The last malaria trial in Ghana was investigated by independence persons.

What is the evidence that there will be strict compliance to the International Committee of Investigators Safety Regulations?

Once you conceive an idea, you write an application, make about 10 copies or 30 depending on requirements by the Food and Drugs Authority. They will then examine the application. On the Ethics Committee there is an attorney (lawyer) and a Reverend Minister. In Kintampo, there are community people on the committee as well.

Our experience with the Food and Drugs Authority Ethics Committee is that they are very thorough. The International Conference on the Formulation of Guidelines uses the criteria described above to assess the information given by Ghana to them. If they are not happy, they can ask us to stop.

FIRST PRESENTATION BY REGULATORS

The moderator Mr Tony Goodman invited the Food and Drugs Authority and the Ghana Health Service to make presentations on the process of approving vaccine trials in Ghana.

Dr Amma Edwin, Ghana Health Service (GHS) Ethics committee

Dr Edwin took participants through the nine points the GHS Ethics Committee uses before giving approval for vaccine trials to be undertaken. She emphasised that in the case of the Ebola trial, none of the processes were short changed. The function of the Committee is to review the information that is submitted to them. The GHS Ethics Committee has 11 members. The committee examines the research protocols to be followed by scientists.

PROTOCOL

Participant recruitment procedures, incentives, language, duration of study and other criteria are supplied on the Information Sheet. There is an adequate opportunity for participants to ask questions and to decide whether to participate or not.

POTENTIAL RISKS

The Information Sheet gives information on any risks and benefits of the study. Incentives should not be seen as too little or too less to encourage people to participate. The Information Sheet must make it clear that participants can withdraw at any time. It must be in a language they understand.

Who to contact; the Information Sheet must provide an address on whom to contact in case of a problem. There must be a telephone number on whom to call at the researcher's office.

Signature; after making the decision, the participant must sign and have a witness who can read and write. After signing the participant can still withdraw at any time.

SECOND PRESENTATION BY REGULATORS

BERNICE LILY DARKO – ACTING DIRECTOR, FOOD AND DRUGS AUTHORITY

She explained that a pre-submission meeting is held with the researchers and investigators. Once a protocol is submitted, the FDA goes through a lot of administrative procedures. The Clinical Trial Department will give their prior approval before a final approval is given.

She explained that if there is no Ethics Committee approval, the FDA will not approve the proposal. Once the trial is approved, there is a monitoring phase when the FDA visits the trial site at least once.

With the Ebola vaccine trial, none of the processes was by-passed. Ethics committees, trial committees, investigators from all the countries were present and the review was facilitated by the WHO. This was the first time this happened in Ghana.

Participating countries visited each other's country and saw the trial sites. Questions were asked by participant countries and answers were given. People were given training about the process.

The FDA has been evaluating trials since 2003. Several Phase 1 and Phase 2 trials have been approved. Ivory Coast and other countries in Africa have been assisted recently by Ghana to review clinical trial applications.

Dr Magda Robalo, WHO Country Representative

She said she only wanted to make six points.

First Point

We have a generational opportunity; this outbreak has been around for 40 years. The only solutions hitherto have been quarantines and isolations. Finding a vaccine against Ebola is therefore an ethical imperative.

Second Point

The unprecedented speed with which participants are taken through trials requires that safety is assured.

There are at least 10 vaccines being developed. The WHO is monitoring the process.

Third Point

The WHO has facilitated and will continue to facilitate Ebola or any other blood disease vaccine trials.

Fourth Point

We have requested Ghana to support sister Africa countries to review clinical trials because Ghana has the expertise in clinical trials. We are grateful to Ghana. We continue to monitor trials; ethics and safety remain paramount. There shall be no wrong doing under our watch.

Fifth Point

Ghana has supported the WHO in research and clinical trials over the years. Ghana's role is critical and is much appreciated.

Sixth Point

We thank Ghanaians; we are monitoring the healthy debate in this country. The most important point is the questions that you will be asking at this forum.

QUESTION TIME

Elizabeth – Africa Media

We are just testing whether the vaccine is safe or not. Is it a safety trial? Are we to understand that the vaccine has no Ebola virus in it? Can we get data in Kenya? Where has Kenya reached in Phase 1 and 2?

Samuel Boateng Arthur – Coalition of NGOs

Is the Ghana Academy of Arts and Sciences here? If they are not here, then after the meeting they will come up with issues again. Were they invited?

Godfred Sey – Rainbow Radio

I want to find out the level of co-operation between the FDA and the MOH. At what point did the Minister realise the problem and put a freeze on the trial?

ANSWERS

PROF BINKA

We have to ensure that the vaccine is safe in human beings. I am on the advisory committee of the trial in Guinea. There are challenges. The CDC trial of experimental vaccines in Liberia and Guinea has been stopped because there is no more an outbreak of Ebola in these countries.

In Sierra Leone, over Six Thousand vaccines have been given already. Without licensing, the Vaccines cannot be given out. It can only be experimental vaccines. Seventy participants were recruited for this same vaccine trial in Oxford, UK and 100 patients in the USA have undergone testing and there are no adverse effects so far. The World Health Organisation (WHO) has made it such that all companies doing the vaccine trial are sharing data.

TONY GOODMAN

We have already held two meetings with the Ghana Academy of Arts and Sciences. We have invited them and every Ghanaian; the invitation is on our social media platform. There is no trial going on in the Volta Region.

FURTHER QUESTIONS

ERIC KOBINA ALONZO; GHANA COALITION OF NGOs

Who is an adult male? Am I healthy? How much are you giving the volunteers?

Daniel Abbey; TV3

At what point did Ghana meet the criteria for the trial?

EVANS YEBOAH, OMAN FM

In Ghana after the work is done you don't hear anything again; how do the volunteers get their money?

PROF WILLIAM AMPOFO, HEAD OF VIROLOGY DEPARTMENT, NOGUCHI LEGON

Looking at the development of the vaccine, I think enough has been done. This is not a full virus; this is a part of the virus that has been engineered to help it generate antibodies in human beings. The Adenovirus is causing respiratory problems and diarrhoea in children. This vaccine trial is happening at an opportune time in Ghana so that the Ministry will have the scientific evidence to make a decision in case of an outbreak. I should remind you that there is also the threat of bird flu. If there is an opportunity we should take part in it. I am worried that Prof Binka is paying GHC200.00 because I am doing a trial and I am paying participants GHC20.00. Next time people will say give me more. Participants have the telephone numbers of the principal investigators. In my research, I have seen telephone call information from study participants asking questions.

DR AMA EDWIN, Ghana Health Service Ethics Committee

A health male adult goes through a medical exam to determine if he is fit to be recruited as a study participant. The Ethics Committee raised the participants' stipend from what the investigators proposed to GHC200.00 per visit to the research site. Subsequent visits attract GHC30.00. Hepatitis B vaccines are also being given. There are the individual level and community level phases of the trial process. How much is being given depends on where you are. You cannot compare the UK to Ghana.

DR MAGDA ROBALO

You have to be committed to be a participant. What you are given makes compensation for transport, time spent, loss of income and other things. The WHO does not define how much participants are paid in each country. Every context is different; they vary from one place to another. The 12 volunteers we are looking for should feel proud of participating in the study. What the WHO will do when all trials are completed is to call scientists from all over the world to agree to move to Phase 3. Whether there is an efficacious vaccine to work on or not is decided at this meeting. I know that from the bottom of your hearts you all want a solution to Ebola. Is it not true? If Ghana is not ready, other countries will go ahead.

The applause Dr Robalo received showed that she hit home right on point. She said the communication gap should be bridged from this meeting. She also said the money should not be an issue but the audience roared in disagreement.

ADDITIONAL QUESTIONS

FREDA ATTEPOR; CONCERNED GHANAIAN

What's in it for Ghana? Does it mean other countries are receiving some compensation?

PROF BINKA

The Ethics Committee decides how much should be given. We have met other countries. Other countries will want to undertake the study but they do not have the capacity. When the outbreak happened some countries did not have the capacity to diagnose it. In the next 12 months, there will be no vaccine for Ebola. The vaccines available can only be called experimental vaccines. When there is an outbreak in Ghana we will have data to show that the experimental vaccine is safe in our population. In the American case, they used experimental vaccines to treat those who were transported there from Liberia. If we have data we stand a good chance of using these experimental vaccines to protect our front line staff. If not which manufacturer will go out of line to release vaccines for an epidemic in Ghana or anywhere it has not been tried?

FREDA ATTEPOR; CONCERNED GHANAIAN

The concerned Ghanaian repeated her question again, seeking to know what's in it for Ghana.

PROF BINKA

It helps us to upgrade our laboratories and medical equipment. Now we have double of every major piece of equipment. The joy for us scientists is that our professional capacity is enhanced, our laboratories are improved and we can go to the manufacturers and recommend what we want.

DR ANTWI AGYEI, FORMER NATIONAL IMMUNISATION MANAGER

The six killer diseases vaccines were tried in other countries; we did not have the capacity in the past to do trials. It means there is enough trust in our scientists now. We do not manufacture vaccines in Ghana. We are looking for an opportunity to manufacture our own vaccines. We don't usually have time to make "*dedey*" on it. I'm sure when the outbreak in West Africa started we all wanted the experimental vaccines to be given if there was an incidence in Ghana even though it was just an experimental vaccine.

NURSE BERNICE YAHYRA, NYAHO MEDICAL CENTRE

What plans do we have for study participants who experience adverse effects? What informed the selection of the study area?

PROF BINKA

Participants are like golden eggs; they have to be followed everyday for one year. We have a system that even after 12 months, they can reach us. We have undertaken to take care of all children who will be born in this area for the next five years. These companies therefore take an insurance policy. We look at the investigators, their experience and qualification. It's by competition. The sites win through competition. This time Kintampo and Hohoe came out tops.

CLOSING REMARKS

TONY GOODMAN

Thank you very much. We are not bringing Ebola into the country. I am glad today we have been able to bring justice to the topic. The Ministry of Health will not allow anyone to manipulate this process.

CHAIRPERSON'S CLOSING REMARKS

DR LINDA VAN OTOO, GREATER ACCRA REGIONAL DIRECTOR, GHANA HEALTH SERVICE

The chairperson acknowledged the presence of the Deputy Director General, Ghana Health Service and the Director of Research, Ghana Health Service who were seated in the middle of the front row.

She said that from today, we hope this matter will be put to rest. Prof Binka will be available to answer questions after the forum. It is better that we ask questions now, she urged.

ANALYSIS AND IMPRESSIONS

The format of the programme has four aspects for consideration. First is the sensitisation of the public to attend the forum. The Ghana Academy of Arts and Sciences received a bashing from participants for not attending. A special invitation should be made to any one of them to attend the next forum. Their endorsement will be very welcoming. We should seek to get them to endorse the public relations efforts. Otherwise some of the speakers at the next forum should be members of the Ghana Academy of Arts and Sciences.

There will always be reactions to vaccine trials in Ghana and everywhere else in the world. The Ministry of Health has a feather in its cap for organising a successful forum; it was so natural and spontaneous. Let us get some chiefs and religious leaders at the next forum. Reactions from the media and the public present at the forum suggested that they had fully understood the issues. As has been said the greatest risk in life is to risk nothing.

Media opinion leaders and radio show hosts should be called into a one-day conference where they will be exposed to the same forum and they will have the time to ask all their questions. The proposed regional tour will be in order. Prof Binka did very well in explaining the issues.

It is expected that since the MOH and the FDA are both government institutions there is the perception that they will cover each other's back. The question of the

US$2,800.00 still lingers. This is because participants were told that the United Kingdom is different from Ghana. Therefore people should not compare what participants received in that country as compensation for volunteering to what participants receive in Ghana.

CLOSING PRAYER

Mr Tony Goodman said the closing prayer at 4:30PM.

PART TWO

A REPORT OF THE EBOLA VACCINE TRIAL PUBLIC FORUM

HELD AT THE KINTAMPO HEALTH RESEARCH CENTRE IN KINTAMPO ON THURSDAY

2ND JULY 2015

EXECUTIVE SUMMARY

This report is the second of national Ebola vaccine trial public fora organised by the Ministry of Health; the first report covers the forum held in Accra. The facts are getting told in simpler and clearer language. There is no experimental Ebola vaccine in Ghana. This is because the Food and Drugs Authority (FDA) has not given approval for the importation of the said vaccine. The FDA approved Phase One of the vaccine trial on June 8, 2015. The Ghana Health Service Ethics Committee, and the Food and Drugs Authority have not yet approved the Phase One trial in Kintampo. This is the reality on the ground. Anyone or any institution that has concerns regarding all the nagging questions has to query the source of the original story - Star FM in Accra. If the original publishers of the vaccine trial story cannot produce the participants who they interviewed or who were given GH200.00, then the professionals should be saved the trouble of answering questions on non-existent facts.

Everywhere there is a Ghana Health Service facility where experimental vaccines would be tried, the Ghana Health Service Ethics Committee would go through the process using the Information Sheet to ensure the right thing has been done. The final approval is however given by the FDA. In Ghana, only 12 participants are to be sampled after male adults have been screened. The Honourable Select Committee of Parliament and all well-meaning Ghanaians should therefore address the 'epidemic of fear' by asking the media to prove where they got their information. The most important assurance however, is that a protein from the virus that caused the epidemic in Congo some 40 years ago has been separated in a laboratory process. This protein has been added to the strain of the Adenovirus which is present in 97% of all the Ebola virus variants as well as the common cold. The experimental vaccine that has been produced therefore is "a picture" of the actual thing; hence the side effect of the experimental vaccine is not the same as the side effect of the Ebola virus disease; they are two different things. What is to be imported into Ghana is therefore not the Ebola virus but a picture of what Ebola will look like by the skilful process of having its protein removed. We are even in a funny situation right now where Kenya has recruited 72 participants, which process was facilitated by Ghanaian scientists. The sponsors, Glaxosmithkline (GSK) can therefore say: 'Thank you, Ghana. See you next time.' This is because about 100 participants have undergone the trial in the United States and similar numbers in the United Kingdom and Switzerland have done the same. Kenya's 72 selected participants are therefore enough for the sponsor. We however have to go ahead because we are a centre of excellence in Africa, training other research centres in the sub-region on behalf of the World Health Organisation. Secondly, "The Ebola virus disease is closer to us and we are all afraid of it, including scientists." We therefore need to be prepared to have an experimental vaccine that in case of any eventuality could be used in our frontline health workers.

The last important thing to remember is that scientific testing centres are not allowed to advertise and announce themselves. During the Cerebrospinal Meningitis (CSM) and malaria vaccine trials, no announcements were made. Yet the vaccines were successfully tested in Kintampo and administered to the extent that for the next 10 years, there is not expected to be any CSM outbreak in Ghana. If anyone should say "But this is Ebola," again the person must be reminded that in post-modern vaccine development, the virus is not knocked down into a comatose state and placed in the vaccine as before; it is a protein in the virus that is taken out and added to something else to create "a perfect mirror image" which is stored in minus 80 degrees of temperature. It therefore loses its efficacy when exposed into our environment. This is one further explanation that the virus and the vaccine are different things altogether. There is therefore no virus in the vaccine and hence no virus will be imported into Ghana when the import permit is finally given. And finally, since there is no import licence yet from the FDA and therefore no experimental vaccine in Ghana, nobody could have been given GHC200 and a mobile phone. The poorest and weakest questions came from media men. They got an equal measure of roars and tongue lashing from participants; they simply do not listen nor pay attention.

WELCOME ADDRESS, DR POKU ASANTE, *Chief Investigator, Kintampo Health Research Centre*

Dr Poku Asante was the MC and moderator of the forum. After the guest speakers and dignitaries had been introduced, Prof Fred Binka, the chief investigator at the Hohoe Health Research Centre and Vice Chancellor of the University of Allied Health Sciences was invited to give an address of the main issues informing the gathering. He was followed by Prof Kwadwo Koram, a scientist from the Noguchi Memorial Institute for Medical Research, University of Ghana, Legon and Dr Amma Edwin, a member of the Ghana Health Service Ethics Committee and Dr Damien Punyire of the Kintampo Health Centre Ethics Review Committee. Their presentations were followed by the question and Answer session. Questions were asked by the chiefs who were seated in the front row as well as media men.

PRESENTATION FROM SCIENTISTS AND INVESTIGATORS

PROF FRED BINKA

WHY ARE WE HERE?

The scientists in Ghana decided to make a contribution to the research on a vaccine against Ebola. More than 10,000 people have died so far. We all thought the disease was going away but now we have a resurgence of the disease. People from Liberia and Guinea are coming to Ghana so we are not safe.

Ghana was selected through competitive bidding. In fact research funds are never awarded freely, you have to compete for it.

I have been personally involved in testing the Meningitis vaccine. The vitamin A and Insecticide Treated Bed nets were tested in a similar way as Ebola. Even the CHPS compound was tested that is why we are rolling it out nationally today.

WHY DO WE NEED THE VACCINE?

The current epidemic is continuing and we need to prepare. One case in Ghana will change the way we live our lives. Nananom, I am sure you will find it very difficult to bury your dead if we have Ebola.

IS THERE A VACCINE?

Currently there is no vaccine. Vaccines are taken through pre clinical trials.

It is tested in mice and chimpanzees. We have come to the end of the pre-clinical phase. The clinical trial has four phases. It is tested in healthy people. About several hundred people are involved. When it is safe, the phase two trial will involve several hundred to thousand people. The dosage is increased at Phase 2. Then come the Phase 3 trial. We see what protections there are during Phase 3. Hundreds and thousands of people are tested. At this stage we are testing for licensure. Millions are then given the vaccine and they are still monitored.

There is no vaccine now. So we have candidate vaccines or experimental vaccines that are being tried. The Phase One trial has been approved to take place in the Hohoe district. There will be a Phase 2 trial in Hohoe and Kintampo but we haven't reached there yet.

WHY WAS HOHOE SELECTED?

The WHO built the Onchocerciasis trial centre in Hohoe some 30 years ago in 1986. It has been successful. The use of Ivermectin around the world to treat Onchocerciasis has benefited from the work done at the Hohoe Health Research Centre.

WHY WAS KINTAMPO SELECTED?

Kintampo is part of the team of elite centres around the world that have been testing vaccines in multi-country studies. Kintampo has done trials for Meningitis and Malaria vaccines. Even though Kintampo is undergoing approval for the Phase Two trial, this current sponsor Johnson and Johnson needs only one site, that is, Hohoe since it needs just 12 study participants. The GSK trial which is Phase Two will take place in both Hohoe and Kintampo.

WHERE HAS THE VACCINE BEEN TESTED IN HUMANS?

Vaccine trial rules require that the manufacturing country is the first place to try it. Hence the medicines have been tried in the US already. The UK, Germany and Switzerland have also done trials. Now Mali, Gabon, Nigeria and Sierra Leone are in various stages of trial processes.

The measles vaccine had the virus weakened. That process is no longer used. Now a vector is used. The common cold is caused by the Adenovirus. What is in the Ebola vaccine is neither Ebola nor common cold. A protein is selected from the genes. The process of selecting the protein is where scientists have their skills.

The vaccines are stored in minus 80 degrees liquid nitrogen. It is so unstable that once the temperature drops, it is useless. There is therefore no need to be afraid of it. GSK's vaccine is a combination of some strains from the chimpanzee Adenovirus and the Ebola glycoprotein.

We are trying to see if humans can develop antibodies to this protein. It is not tested on sick people. Side effects may include physical pain, tiredness, fever and general lethargy. However, these side effects are only side effects of the experimental vaccine, not side effects of Ebola Virus Disease.

SELECTION OF PARTICIPANTS

We screened 500 people to find 12 people. Most of us will fail these tests. Those who pass are given a chance to participate.

WILL CHILDREN BE TESTED?

Yes but first we must try it in adults.

WILL PREGNANT WOMEN TAKE PART?

No. In all vaccine trials, pregnant women are excluded.

ARE VOLUNTEERS PAID?

No. Participants are however compensated for their time.

WHAT IS THE ACT AUTHORISING THESE TRIALS?

An Act of Parliament has authorised the Food and Drugs Authority to do what it is doing. Also the Ethics Committee looks at the study and ensures that scientists follow principles of justice. The Guinea pigs, if there are any, are therefore the Americans and Europeans who were first recruited into the trials as study participants.

WHY DON'T YOU EDUCATE PEOPLE BEFORE STARTING?

This is the crux of the matter? We are not allowed to advertise. We got approval only on June 8, 2015 and the media problems started. In previous trials, we did not announce a trial. We forgot that this is a political disease. From June 8, 2015 we needed to recruit 12 participants and there was no time to do a media campaign even if we wanted to.

WHEN WILL WE KNOW THE RESULTS?

We will not know the results until all the participating countries have submitted their results and the results have been compiled.

WHEN WILL WE HAVE A VACCINE?

There is no vaccine. Only a candidate or experimental vaccine is what is being tried.

PROF KWADWO KORAM, *Noguchi Memorial Institute For Medical Research*

The chairman of the Parliamentary Select Committee felt there was no need to discuss the matter on the floor of the House.

We are afraid of Ebola disease like anybody else. When there is a vaccine we look at those who got it and those who did not get the disease and they are given vaccines to see how people will react. That stage in the trial of a vaccine is done in a country where there is an outbreak. Such a trial is not being done yet because there is no vaccine.

WILL THE VACCINES WORK IN PEOPLE WITH EBOLA?

The best way in the past was to take the virus and take it through a test which disables it from causing diseases. That era is gone. No more licences are given for such experiments.

Currently we examine the organism and look at which parts of it can cause disease. We create a picture of the organism.

The part which is common to all the viruses (strains) is taken together with the parts of the virus which caused the disease in Congo 40 years ago.

When you go to the Food and Drugs Authority you have to show which animal, male or female was used in the experiment. The experimental vaccine showed complete success in animals hence the approval has been given for trials in humans.

It has also been shown that the common cold virus whose parts are being used are incapable of causing any other disease in humans.

If your vaccine has the same symptoms as the disease, no one will buy it. So why will anyone make a vaccine which produces symptoms of the very disease it seeks to prevent.

GAAS said there was prolonged bleeding in some trial cases. These are true but these people recovered within a week without having taken in any medicine.

For those who experienced bleeding, there was a drop in the number of cells that help blood clot but the number of cells went back up to normal levels within a week.

MRS YVONNE ADU BOAHEN, *Food & Drugs Authority (FDA)*

We encourage face to face meetings with investigators before they bring their application.

It takes about 15 working days to process the application. The application includes the protocol. The review committee will look at the application and examine the work of all the units involved. Then there must be an ethics approval from the Ethics Committee. The application is then passed when appropriate. The FDA also monitors the trial process.

Phase 1 was approved on June 8, 2015 and the Phase 2 application is still pending.

The US FDA, Health Canada, European Medicine Agency and Ghana FDA were organised by the WHO to facilitate the process of application and what needs to be done.

The sponsor then answered questions and the GHS Ethics committee also got answers to questions. The FDA's 12-member committee also gave their responses.

The FDA went to inspect the trial sites and made sure standards were met at both national and international levels.

The International Committee on Harmonisation Protocol Guidelines for Clinical Trials E6RI was followed. The FDA has qualified staff that are even hired by WHO to supervise trials in other countries.

The FDA has been recognised as a regional centre of excellence for clinical trials. The FDA uses this status to supervise other trials around Africa and to give training and support to other African countries. This shows that the FDA is way ahead. A prophet may however not be welcome in his own hometown.

DR AMMA EDWIN, *Ghana Health Service (GHS), Ethics Review Committee.*
Her presentation focused on participant involvement in clinical trials. We look out for the interest of participants.

The GHS Ethics Committee has been tasked to ensure that anytime there is a trial being done in a GHS facility, there will be a review and inspection. We had pertinent concerns which were addressed at the forum organised by the WHO. Our concern is that study participants understand what they are going into. We ensure informed consent. We use the Information Sheet and the Consent Form.

Sometimes people may confuse a vaccine trial (research) with diseased people being given medicine. We explain this to them. We also look at benefits.

The GHS Ethics Committee ensured that the Hepatitis B vaccine will be given as part of the trial and this was incorporated by the WHO.

Compensation was also determined. What the sponsors initially offered was too low and would take advantage of people. The GHC200.00 that you have heard about was decided by the GHS Ethics Committee. There is also international insurance. The Ethics Committee makes sure that the research has insurance. If you get sick as a participant during the study period, there is provision to take care of you. It is a full international insurance. All this information regards the Hohoe trial. The Kintampo trial has not yet been approved by the GHS Ethics Committee. If you choose to take part and you want to stop, you can stop at any time.

DR DAMIEN PUNYIRE, *Kintampo Health Research Centre Ethics Committee.*
Our role is to look at the local context within which this research is to take place. This committee has renowned researchers, human and children's rights activists, chiefs and clinicians.

Sometimes we review protocols from other places. We review the scientific protocol; the science of it and the ethics of it. There are international guidelines that protect subjects or study participants. All those are reviewed. We discuss both known and potential risks and benefits. At all times the benefits must be far greater than the risks. The compensation and informed consent firms are also studied. We give rejection, conditional approval or full acceptance. The application came around 8 April 2015 and the process was followed. Approval is not a guarantee for investigators to work independently. We work hand in hand with them.

QUESTIONS AND ANSWERS

NANA OWUSU PINKRAH II, *Krontihene of Kintampo Nwoase*

Initially I was confused listening to the radio but now I've got educated by medical minds. There is the perception that the virus was a laboratory mistake and others also have it that it was a plan to wipe out the black race in Africa among other conspiracy theories. Why is the vaccine trial not being conducted in Ebola-hit countries like Liberia and Sierra Leone? What happened to the Swiss when they were introduced to the vaccine trial?

Answer: PROF BINKA

10,000 people have died and health workers have gone down with the disease. Nobody is able to do the Phase Two trial where there is exposure because the disease is there; these trials are done in healthy populations.

Yes even if it was a conspiracy theory or a laboratory mistake as they say about HIV conspiracy theories my approach is that what can we do? We all have to do something now that it is here. There is a stage where the vaccine is tried in areas suffering outbreaks. This is not a vaccine so we cannot try it in outbreak zones. This is an experimental vaccine and so it must be tried in healthy populations. That is the rule by international standards. We cannot afford not to do anything. When your neighbour's beard is on fire, you have to put yours in water.

Answer: PROF KORAM

There is the epidemic of disease and there is the epidemic of fear. The conspiracy theories are there but you cannot get anybody to prove that to you. We are not going to test the virus but rather the vaccine. It is a very serious disease and nobody wants to get close to it. There was one doctor who treated a patient. He then felt some itches on his forehead and scratched it. And that was it. He was gone. So why would anyone want to go and bring the virus here? The vaccine does not give you the same symptoms as the virus itself. When we get to Phase 3 and there is no disease in the population we cannot use it or try it there. One of the problems of the H1N1 flu vaccine trials was that it did not go through the phases of this vaccine and there were reports of people collapsing but this trial will be a different story. Up until now, in the early case in Congo, about 400 cases occurred and some 220 died.

The early cases of Ebola recorded in Uganda were in the hundreds in rural areas but this time around they were in the urban areas, thereby killing thousands of people. I say when Ebola arrives in Ghana we'll all see it because of the way the disease occurs.

The Swizz were given the vaccines and the symptoms were pains in your arms and a few other symptoms. Nobody has been given the vaccine and died. The conspiracy theories exist but when you hear them, question them.

Question: BEDIMAA DUUT, *Municipal Health Director, Goaso*
I want to get the material to educate our people.

Answer: DR OWUSU AGYEI
The material is available for assembly men and community people but listen first.

Question: NANA AGYEI ADINKRA II, *Krontihene Of Mo Traditional Area*

How does one become a participant?

Answer: PROF BINKA

There has to be testing. If any of your body systems does not meet the criteria, you are not allowed to participate.

Answer: PROF KORAM

If we test in a country with the disease how do we know these are the people who have it and those who do not because Ebola collapses the health system? You can't use countries with the disease because it's very difficult to differentiate the sick from the healthy people.

Question: ANTWI BOASIAKO, *Classic FM, Techiman*.

How were communities educated in Hohoe? Were mobile phones distributed?

Answer: PROF BINKA

All these questions were manufactured by the press. As we speak, the vaccines have not arrived in the country. When the approval comes, you have to apply for a permit to import the vaccines into the country. My wife is Charity Binka who was a journalist for many years. So she saw that the media were making mistakes. Star FM described me as the Pro Vice Chancellor but I am the Vice Chancellor.

Question: PASTOR HAYFORD ASANTE, *ICGC, Local Council of Churches*

What are the benefits to the community? What are the measures that were taken?

Answer: PROF KORAM

There is no trial going on. I am surprised that the media said we've gone to nursing schools to administer it on midwives. We don't even have approval to import the vaccines into the country.

Answer: DR OWUSU AGYEI

In the previous trials, we got insurance that covered six years.

Answer: DR. KOFI ISSAH, *Deputy Director of Public Health, Brong Ahafo*

In 2012, we finally vaccinated the three Northern Regions against CSM. For the next 10 years, if people stay healthy no one will get CSM. Why don't you interview the so-called participants of Hohoe? Now the journalists are saying they can't find the participants who they claim they interviewed?

Answer: PROF BINKA

Some lady said we were doing trials in Navrongo. We sued the lady but since 2009 the case is still in court. If we were to get justice quickly, these false reports would stop.

Question: MICHAEL EFFAH, *Dinpa FM, Sunyani.*

I want to know the insurance package after the vaccine trial. The lay man may think that if it's a government policy and there is a change of government, he won't get the compensation.

The audience roared that it's not a government policy.

Answer: DR AMMA EDWIN

If there is an outbreak the community who went through the trial will benefit first from the vaccination.

Answer: PROF BINKA

We started Universities in Hohoe and Brong Ahafo and within three years, our university in Hohoe is conducting a vaccine trial. Professionals are calling from all over the world and are saying if you guys are doing this already then I'm coming back home. We are scientists and we also want to lead in research, what is wrong with that?

Question: IBN DAOUD, *Ghana Health Service, Kintampo*

What is the way forward? When these reactions came, we did not hear Ghana Health Service or the investigators or the FDA. We left it to the politicians to defend it. Secondly can you get a word to replace the word TRIAL?

Question: NANA AKUA, *Asta FM*

What is the age group who can take part in the trial? Does the protocol precede the trial? Does the Ethics Committee approval come before FDA approval?

Answer: DR POKU ASANTE

The word TRIAL is an international term and we can't change it to deceive people by avoiding the use of the word trial. The protocol is part of the process. The age group is adults 18-55 years. If the vaccine is safe, an independent group of scientists from around the world will give approval to the next age group which is children. You need the Ethics Committee approval before the FDA approval. If the FDA approves and the Ethics Committee disapproves later, then you have deceived the public. So the final approval comes from the FDA.

Answer: PROF. BINKA

Ghana and Kenya were to recruit at the same time. Kenya has recruited 72 participants. This is a competitive recruitment process. Ghana was helping to recruit people in Guinea, Sierra Leone, Kenya and other places. Yet when it comes to Ghana people are undermining the process. The sponsor has really bent over backwards because they have already got their 72 participants so they might as well say thank you Ghana see you next time. All this while that Kenya is ready, Ghana is still going through the FDA and GHS approval processes.

CLOSING REMARKS

MR JUSTICE MCHAEL BAFFOE, *Municipal Chief Executive, Kintampo North*

He summarised the day's proceedings and urged that an exclusive session for the media should be organised.

ANALYSIS AND IMPRESSIONS

The principal task of this ongoing public engagement on the experimental vaccine trial against Ebola in Ghana is the need to demystify the fears of citizens. From the questions that were given it was clear that people do not understand the message, especially journalists and media men. This report recommends that this must be considered.

This is simple for anybody on the street to think about but it is not true when it comes to vaccine trials. The reactions from the journalists and participants at the forum, during the Questions and Answer session showed that they did not grab the message. The Kintampo North Municipal Chief Executive (MCE), from this background, suggested to the Ministry of Health to organise a forum specifically on the education of journalists. He observed that once they understand the subject matter, there is a greater likelihood that it will trickle down to the people.

The presence of the Chiefs was a very important addition to the forum. Their questions were very good. This should be repeated at other fora. The speakers spoke with more confidence and they should be encouraged to continue in that manner. One cannot think of any bad thing they said which could be used against them or which could create a public relations crisis for the Ministry of Health.

PART THREE

A REPORT OF THE EBOLA VACCINE TRIAL PUBLIC FORUM

HELD AT THE NAVRONGO HEALTH RESEARCH CENTRE IN NAVRONGO ON FRIDAY

3RD JULY 2015

EXECUTIVE SUMMARY

The Navrongo forum is highly recommended by all participants. The Navrongo Health Research Centre in Ghana has produced a lot of scientists including Prof Fred Binka.

Prof Binka is a renowned researcher and lead investigator of many vaccine trials in Ghana. That is the news story. Prof Binka led the research that found vaccines for Onchocerciasis, Insecticide Treated Bed Nets, The Community Health and Planning Services (CHPS) compounds. And he would not have been what he is today without the training he got at the "University of Navrongo Health Research Centre as he jokingly called the centre. The fact that independent analysts and people from all backgrounds were looking for a photo opportunity with him is also the news story. We can ride on the back of Prof Binka to kill the debate. That's a fact. And he also has a passion to see this through. A vaccine for Ebola would be a crowning moment for him. And why not? As was declared by one of the speakers, every Member of Parliament is seeking to get to the top. Scientists also want to get to the top. What's wrong with that? To cut a long story short, the forum was held at the conference room of the Prof Fred Binka Building.

The arguments are reduced to two main issues. One is the rise of Prof Binka. Two is the bad publicity media men at the various fora are giving themselves. They would not listen. And they will continue to ask silly questions even seconds after that same question has been answered. Prof Binka is however more charitable. He spares the media and chides the Ghana Academy of Arts and Sciences (GAAS) for making this matter a debate in the "papers". "Scientific cannot exist without debate," he declared. However such debate is not done in the papers as the GAAS has done. He also contended that they, the scientists, are not the best placed people to handle communication but some contributors disagreed with him. And the audience agreed. "The man has got his stuff right: "If we face the epidemic today the health system cannot cope. We also do not have the protection against the disease for our front line health workers." By WHO standards, a vaccine will not be approved in less than 24 months. If we conduct this trial, we can have an experimental vaccine that in case of any outbreak, we can ask the manufacturers to produce for us at a very good negotiated price because we have tried the experimental vaccine in our healthy population.

In a photo opportunity in front of the Fred Binka Building he said quietly to the communication team from the MOH, Accra that a prophet is not welcome in his own home. The team had commented in awe that they were standing in front of a building named after him. The rep of the Ethics Review Committee of the Ghana Health service, Dr Amma Edwin remarked at the forum that she had attended the fora in Parliament, Accra, Kintampo and Navrongo but this Navrongo forum is the best. The PR team however noticed one big flaw; the absence of Dr Poku Asante, Director of the Kintampo Health Research Centre. He had no reason to be absent. He must get into his usual role as moderator or Master of Ceremony. The man is so good at debating the issue.

WELCOME ADDRESS, DR ABRAHAM ODURO, *Director, Navrongo Health Research Centre*

The meeting started with an opening prayer at 10:00AM.

Dr Abraham Oduro, Director of Navrongo Health Research Centre was the MC and moderator. He said the Ebola virus is the most deadly virus in recent times. We need information on the way forward.

Dr Oduro introduced the Chairman, Dr Kwaku Awoonor Williams, the Upper East Regional Director of the Ghana Health Service. The chairman in accepting the chair remarked that the Ebola Virus Disease is not a new disease. He further explained that we have about 17 borders out of the Upper East Region. We must therefore work hard to address the problem.

PRESENTATION FROM SCIENTISTS AND INVESTIGATORS

PROF FRED BINKA

Prof Binka said he attended the "University of Navrongo" Health Research Centre and that is what has made him the expert that he is today. He mentioned his topic and also said what the other speakers are to do. The epicentre in West Africa has experienced about 25,000 cases and 10,000 deaths across three countries, he explained. From our knowledge the disease still rages on. If we face the epidemic today the health system cannot cope. We also do not have the protection against the disease for our front line health workers who will treat the cases.

A vaccine is important because it protects people against diseases. That is why we have a solid BCG vaccine that protects children against diseases.

IS THERE A VACCINE?

No. And there won't be a vaccine for the next 24 to 36 months. This makes what we are going to do today very important.

First trials were carried out in laboratories in chimpanzees and they were shown to be protective in those animals. But what is protective in animals may not be protective in humans. So Phase 1 involves injecting 20 to 100 healthy adults with the virus construct to see how people will react. When you have a disease, that small vaccine is not going to make any difference because you already have the disease.

The second stage involves trying it on more people and increasing the dosage. Here too it is done in healthy adults. Then at stage three we try it in more people, not necessarily healthy adults, you try it in the general population.

The fourth stage is done before you apply for a licence. You try in more people. Even after licence, the vaccine can be withdrawn if it creates problems. In Ghana, we are trying Phase 1 by Johnson and Johnson and the Phase 2 trial will be by GlaxoSmithKline (GSK).

WHY HOHOE?

Hohoe is the first place in Ghana where a phase 1 trial was started. The Onchocerciasis vaccine was tested in Hohoe and Ivermectin together with other combination medicines was developed against the small worm that causes Onchocerciasis.

Mali, Kenya, Burkina Faso, Guinea and Nigeria are doing the same trials. Ghana is ahead not behind. The rotor studies were done here, Malaria bed nets and so on and they were successful. We are not guinea pigs. Ghana, Mali, Kenya and Uganda are doing this now.

We all get cold. The viruses of the common cold are taken and the genes are knocked out. So it is no more common cold. Then the protein from the Ebola virus is added to the cold virus. Then you develop a vector, not a virus. Some scientists say they will not use the virus that causes diseases in humans (Human flu virus) but the Chimpanzee Adenovirus and then the protein from the Ebola virus is added to this vector. Therefore the virus that is selected cannot cause disease in humans because they are from chimpanzees. However, it offers us protection from the Ebola virus because it produces antibodies that fight the Ebola virus. How you select the protein will determine whether you're a drug manufacturer or not.

HOW DO YOU RECRUIT PEOPLE?

Over 500 people will be screened but only 12 will be selected. We screen people for lipid levels, hypertension and many others. It is tried in adults, healthy male adults. We do not know if it is safe in children because we have not reached there yet. Pregnant women are not allowed in vaccine trials just as in drugs trials. On the 2nd February, 2015 Hohoe applied for trials to be done and it got approval on June 8. It is not in a rush. We were to recruit 72 participants between Ghana and Kenya. Kenya got its approval on 8 March 2015 and recruited all the 72 whilst Ghanaians are still doing public education. After the approval is given a contract will be signed between the sponsors and the Centre. What we are doing is backed by the Public Health Act passed by Parliament. When I was growing up, there were more churches in Liberia than anywhere else on the West Coast of Africa! So Christians you can pray but allow the scientists to work. Nobody knows why the disease came to Liberia despite their prayers.

If we allow this process to go on, we shall have an experimental vaccine within the next 2 years. Second, we have the human capacity to do it. If you are a parliamentarian, you want to get to the top. We scientists also want to get to the top. Why are we not hailing our scientists that they have been able to bring this contract here to Ghana?

DR ABRAHAM ODURO, *Director, Navrongo Health Research Centre*.
Dr Oduro took the opportunity to respond to the questions which were raised by the Ghana Academy of Arts and Sciences (GAAS) and others.

He said some persons wanted to know if pre-clinical trials had been done in animals first. He explained that it was first tried in animals and now in humans. He explained that it is expected that the virus will not change its form since the vector that has been captured in the vaccine has about 97% of the characteristics of all the various strains of Ebola. If the virus changes, then we will have to go back to the drawing board and start with new vaccine research and trials. Dr Oduro was not good at delivering the Question & Answer Session where a prepared text of responses is delivered in response to the Ghana Academy of Arts and Sciences and others. Dr Opoku Asante from the Kintampo Health Research Centre should come back and do that job. Dr Oduro spoke too fast and so he did not make an impression through the speakers.

DR AMMA EDWIN, *Ghana Health Service (GHS), Ethics Review Committee*

The GHC 200.00 in the media was approved by the GHS Ethics Review Committee. It also recommended that the Hepatitis B vaccine should be given in addition to this experimental vaccine. We also look at the insurance package before we allow the consent form to be signed. Participants are given the forms to go home and read it. The telephone number of the administrator of the GHS Ethics Review Committee is given to study participants to call at anytime they have queries.

There is a test of understanding in English, Ewe and Twi to make sure that the participants really understand what they are doing. After the test and the consent form you can still withdraw from the trial if you no longer feel like taking part.

ZAKARIA BRAIMAH, *Regional Officer, Food and Drugs Authority (FDA)*

The process of approval is lengthy. This application got approved in about 4 months. We have a maximum period of 60 days to approve the clinical trials. A flow diagram illustrates how the work is organised. I do not know why this one took longer. If there are no queries, then the application is approved. If an application is rejected, the applicant may appeal to the Minister of Health within 60 days.

QUESTIONS AND ANSWERS

Question: EDWARD ADISI, *Metro TV Regional Correspondent*

We in the media will give all the support needed. Now our honourable Prof Binka said we are looking at healthy adults. In a crowd of 20 people how we do get the people who meet the criteria? Are we going to reduce the criteria or extend the time frame? Let us use leadership by example. I'm glad that our chiefs are also here. Let us get our parliamentarians to volunteer. They are in both NDC and NPP.

Question: PAULINA TINDAANA, *Navrongo Health Research Centre*

First of all I want to commend the Ministry of Health for organising this forum to educate us and allay the fears of Ebola being introduced in this country. I would like to use this opportunity to encourage our leaders to make public engagement a priority. They must do public engagement before starting this research. Our scientists must have strong stakeholders' engagement. Is this the case that participants will be given mobile phones?

Question: RAYMOND ALLOU, *Regional NDC Rep & Assembly Member*

You in the media, leave NDC and NPP out. Let's tackle this Ebola fear and panic among the masses and not meddle in politics for now. When the election draws near in 2016, then we will talk about politics. Thank you.

Question: ASIBI BANGUU-EKELLE, *GBC, URA Radio, Bolgatanga*

Communication is key. Communication is everything. Occasionally NDC and NPP may come but Ebola is more dangerous and more threatening than anything.

Question: DR EVELYN SAKEAH, *Navrongo Health Research Centre*

Is there a compensation for those who will die or have disabilities in the event of the vaccine trial?

Question: AHMED NAEEM, *WRCL*

When it comes to leadership by example, the theory collapses on its head because even if leaders volunteer they have to be screened and they may not meet the criteria.

Answer: PROF BINKA

If somebody at the border gets quarantined, samples get taken to Noguchi and the epidemiologist calls the Regional Director in Bolgatanga that the sample confirms Ebola, then you will understand what we are talking about preparation. We must all prepare. We cannot relax the criteria. We get a few people. The criterion is strict so that the results you get can be generalised.

We were trying to recruit 36 people originally in Hohoe. We never thought of mounting a public education because it is against the law. If we are doing a vaccine trial in Navrongo we do not go to Bawku to talk about it. We have learnt our lessons, the FDA has learnt its lessons and everyone has recognised the need to do a public campaign next time.

We scientists are not the best people to handle communication. We have also learnt what is bad about communication. If the Ghana Academy of Art and Sciences have a problem about a study in Hohoe, they must call the scientists and debate it. They should not write to the papers and do a media reaction. In fact science without debate will not be science. In fact, parliament has told us to avoid the debate in the papers and debate among ourselves. As for the political issues, I agree that the media should look at some of the issues that affect our daily lives and talk about them.

Answer: DR AMMA EDWIN

The GHS Ethics Review Committee gave approval on 16 April 2015 and the FDA gave approval on 8 June and by the rules the investigators could not have gone public with it. Dr Edwin agreed with Paulina that the stakeholders must lead the campaign.

PROF BINKA

In Zaire 100 people died, Prof Peter Piers was sent by his professor in Belgium to go and investigate some so-called strange deaths in Zaire. He was then a PhD student. He is still alive and he has been visiting Ghana regularly. Later in Uganda, 400 people died. Why was there no attention then? Does any journalist here know of any organisation which has sponsored any malaria drug or vaccine? he asked.

There was no answer. "Most of the anti-malaria drugs were funded by the US Military because no manufacturer wanted to fund it," he explained.

Ebola has become prominent because 10,000 people have died. When the US citizens got infected, they carried them one plane per infected case. There could be conspiracy theories. I do not have the means to doubt that but some of us are also interested in finding solutions. Why stop me? Why deny me my right to save human lives? When Ghana participates, the manufacturers and companies doing the trials cannot determine the price alone. In the case of the rotor virus trial, because communities participated in it, it now costs about $5 and we even have it for free. By all means we can create our conspiracy theories but allow us to continue our research.

Answer: DR AMMA EDWIN

In Congo last august about 70 infections occurred and 43 people died, more than half. Why the interest now. Ebola is an orphan disease. There are certain diseases that commercial interests will never fund. Let us think globally because if we focus so much on the conspiracy theories we will never find solutions. I have participated in the forum in Accra, Kintampo and Navrongo. This is the one I have enjoyed the most. You journalists are so powerful. Do not be the first to put out wrong information. We now have an epidemic of fear caused by journalists.

DR ABRAHAM ODURO

The speakers have to drive to Tamale and catch a flight to Accra so we really need to end here. This comment could have been avoided since the people were already convinced. It creates the impression that the organisers are running away from the questions. Meanwhile it was announced that Prof Binka world be available to questions.

CLOSING REMARKS

DR AWOONOR WILLIAMS, *Upper East Regional Director of Ghana Health Service*

He made the audience laugh by narrating a story of a bus of some 50 people at the Paga border who were coming from Guinea. This bus had been turned away from the Ivory Coast border. National Security, Regional Minister and everybody was refusing to answer phone calls or giving excuses. Nobody wanted to go to the spot and make a decision. Eventually the bus was turned away. Meanwhile the Customs and Immigration Officers were sitting down collecting their passports, exchanging pleasantries, shaking hands and going about their jobs in usual fashion. He concluded therefore that the fears are real. Closing remarks were given at 12:39PM.

ANALYSIS AND IMPRESSION

The Navrongo forum was geared towards engaging the general public into the advocacy for the Ebola vaccine trial to be conducted in Ghana. The forum received massive attendance by the general public, more especially the chiefs and political leaders of Navrongo. There was also the presence of some Senior High School students in the Navrongo township. It was a great spectacle to see the renowned researcher and lead investigator, Prof Binka give a heartfelt statement about how he started his career as a researcher in the Navrongo Health Research Centre much to the delight of the audience, especially members of the Navrongo Health Research Centre. The presence of the Chiefs and the Senior High School children added a new colour to the function. The Question and Answer session proved to be very educational and the common feature was the need to discard playing political games with the trial process. More members of the public should be encouraged to attend such conferences to broaden the debate.

Just like the idea that the death of a relative is not my own death, Ghanaians simply think that they are exempted from the Ebola Virus Disease. The danger when a nation begins to think like this is that the nation may bury more people when it least expects it.

Members of the Navrongo Traditional Council were there to grace the occasion with their authoritative presence.

They were:

Arthur Wekem Baliana Adda	-	Navrongo
Batabi Tiyiamu,	-	Kayoro
Ayikude Zamgyeo	-	Katiu
Peter Asanchera Alua	-	Kazigu

We are really grateful for their regal presence.

PART FOUR

A REPORT OF THE EBOLA VACCINE TRIAL FORUM

HELD AT THE PENSIONERS' HALL IN HO

ON MONDAY 6TH JULY 2015

EXECUTIVE SUMMARY

The breaking news about the planned commencement of an Ebola vaccine trial in Ghana created considerable concern, panic and anxiety amongst the citizens.

The Minister for Health was summoned to Parliament. There, the consensus was that the planned trial was ill-advised and there had not been enough public education.

Consequently, the trial was deferred until the concerns of stake-holders had been addressed.

As part of this process, a public forum was held in Ho at which the general public and the media were invited to interact with resource persons involved directly and indirectly with various aspects of the trial.

The resource persons were Prof Fred Binka, Dr Amma Edwin, Delese Mimi Darko and Prof Kwadwo Koram.

The main areas of contention were as follows;

1. What is a clinical trial?

2. What is the exact component of the vaccine to be injected?

3. What is the legal and regulatory framework governing the initiation and conduct of a clinical trial and have these been followed?

4. Why has Ghana chosen to participate?

5. What benefits will accrue to Ghana?

6. Who will participate as the trial subjects and how will they be chosen?

7. What dangers if any will the subjects and the general population face?

8. What measures and resources have been put in place to eliminate or minimise these dangers?

9. What is the quantum of money that will be paid to the trial subjects and how does this compare to figures from Europe and America and why the difference if any?

It was agreed that Ghana needed to participate in the global effort to find an Ebola Vaccine. There are potential benefits for our educational, health and economic system.

Evidence was also provided that Ghana had the internationally recognised institutions, the personnel and the legal framework to perform clinical trials in order to test and discover new drugs and vaccines.

The debate as to the appropriateness of the trial bordered on three questions, namely; adherence to laid down procedures, transparency and public education.

With respect to these questions, the resource persons explained the legal framework and the required procedures. They insisted that these had been painstakingly adhered to.

A detailed attempt was made to address the comprehensive technical questions that had been posed by the Ghana Academy of Arts and Sciences.

The public was assured that there was no chance of the Ebola virus replicating and infecting any member of the study group or the general population.

It was emphasised that the study population will be monitored closely and any adverse medical reactions treated promptly.

With the benefit of hindsight, the researchers surmised that they should have been more proactive and forthcoming with information above and beyond the routine amounts provided for other clinical trials such as malaria and rotor virus.

Finally, it was agreed that there should be capacity building with respect to communication in science in order to prevent a recurrence of the above situation.

WELCOME ADDRESS, DR JOSEPH NUETEY, *Regional Director of the Ghana Health Service*

The programme started at 10:30AM. Miss Afua Djansi Asamoah, Public Relations Officer of the Ghana Health Service, Ho was the Master of Ceremony. She introduced the guests, Dr Joseph Nuetey, Regional Director of the Ghana Health Service as the Chairman. Prof Kwadwo Koram, a scientist from the Noguchi Memorial Institute for Medical Research, University of Ghana, Legon and Dr Amma Edwin, a member of the Ghana Health Service Ethics Committee, Dr Abraham Hodgeson, Director of Research, Ghana Health Service and Miss Delese Mimi Darko, an Acting Director Food and Drugs Authority (FDA).

WELCOME ADDRESS, DR JOSEPH NUETEY, *Regional Director of the Ghana Health Service*

As you all know this is a very important exercise. We have all talked about it in our bedrooms and those who have the courage have said it openly. We have come to discuss it as it should be. If you liken it to somebody climbing a flight of stairs, we can say we have missed a step, and we have tumbled. Something went wrong and so there was hue and cry. I do not know if there has been a precedent. But what I know is that clinical trials have gone on in this country for years without much issue.

We in the Volta Region accept the vaccine trial. We have now got the opportunity to add our name to the list of places. This clinical trial has scared everybody to the spine. From the scientific perspective nobody should get Ebola disease from this vaccine trial. There is no way a glycoprotein taken from one virus and placed in another virus should give you a disease.

We had a very bad experience last week when some of our immunisation officers went into the villages for immunisation and the mothers rushed to collect their children. So we know that some damage has been caused by this publicity. We should all participate and ask questions. Enjoy the forum.

PRESENTATION FROM SCIENTISTS AND INVESTIGATORS

PROF FRED BINKA, *Vice Chancellor, University of Health and Allied Sciences (UHAS*)

This is a very important day in the life of the University of Allied Health Sciences. I must thank the Minister of Health for this opportunity. We have been to four Regions and we have two more to go.

A group of us came together and decided that this was an opportunity to investigate this disease. Where we are geographically, this disease is close to us. Among the candidate vaccines, we felt that this experimental vaccine being proposed could provide a way out. Through the work of the Noguchi Memorial Institute for Medical Research Hohoe and Kintampo were selected. We were chosen to be part of a competitive multi-country study.

WHY DO WE NEED THE VACCINE?

If you have travelled through the Ebola region, people are fighting this disease with only their clothes on. One of the best ways of fighting the disease is to make sure you do not get the disease at all. To make things worse there are no vaccines approved, only some experimental vaccines. There will be no vaccines licensed in the next 48 months.

The vaccines we have in our EPI system are given to children from birth when their mothers go to the immunisation centres.

The vaccines are tested in mice and chimpanzees and when they are successful then we test in humans. The animal vaccine trial always precedes the human trial. The human trial has four phases.

Our goal in Phase One is to find out if the vaccine is safe in humans. About 20 to 100 people are tested. We go to Phase Two and try it in more people making sure the vaccine is safe. In Phase Three we increase the number of participants and find out if it is 30% safe or 50% safe. But the main goal is to test that it is efficacious. When the results are safe we apply to the licensing authority. Then we go to Phase Four where we can use the vaccine in an epidemic.

WHY WAS HOHOE SELECTED?

The Onchocerciasis Research Centre in Hohoe has done more than 30 trials in the past 30 years. It has worked with the Noguchi Memorial Institute for Medical

Research and other institutions. The University of Health and Allied Sciences is poised to take over from the Hohoe Onchocerciasis Centre. Kintampo also met the same criteria. The US, UK and Switzerland have Phase One trials in their healthy population.

Mali, Gabon and Kenya have started and have concluded the Phase One trials. Johnson and Johnson and GSK have met the criteria of identifying the strains of Ebola that are multiplying. The vaccine being tested has 97% of all the strains' characteristics. The candidate vaccine is called a construct. People who receive it will have fever, cold and headache but the good news is that these side effects go away after a short while. Our goal is to find out if there are any unknown side effects.

The participants will go through a thorough screening process. Healthy adults 18 to 55 years are tested. If we find it safe in adults, then children could be tried. Further studies could be done to see if it is safe in pregnant women but they are always the last.

Volunteers are not paid. Some compensation is paid but it is not a job for which you should get money.

You should express an interest in the sponsor. Visit the study sites, have meetings and then you the centre will apply to the Food and Drugs Authority. After completing the protocols then you get approval but they will be with you throughout the process. The same application documents are submitted to the GHS National Ethics Review Committee.

LEGAL FRAMEWORK

What happened after a licence is akin to what happens when you take your case to court. You cannot talk about the cause when it is being tried because you will have problems with the judge. The lesson we have learnt is that while we cannot talk about it, the media is talking about it. But they must be fair to all sides of the story. This multi-country study is now being done in Sierra Leone as well.

WHAT ARE THE BENEFITS?

In case of an epidemic, we can use those experimental vaccines in our population. The trials are going on right now in Burkina Faso, Mali, Kenya, Uganda and Tanzania. I beg your pardon. I think Ghana must be on that list. Thank you very much.

RESPONSES TO GHANA ACADEMY OF ARTS AND SCIENCES (GAAS) QUESTIONS

PROF KWADWO KORAM, *Noguchi Memorial Institute for Medical Research, Legon*

We have been to see the Parliamentary Select Committee on Health. They felt that since the GAAS is the august body of science we needed to respond to them.

Nobody certainly knows how a transmission occurs. There are stories about hunters who bring game and in the process of preparation get sick, go to hospital and it spreads. Up until now it occurred in East African forests and in small numbers of people so nobody gave it a serious thought. There are stories this morning of some hunters killing antelopes and getting infected but now all six have tested negative to Ebola disease. So nobody knows exactly how it occurs.

People say experiments go wild in the lab, but in this case nobody has said that some experiments have gone wild. But if some experiments have gone wild do we fold our arms and do nothing? This protein has 97% of the characteristics of all the strains of Ebola.

Vaccine production is not a spell-of-the-moment issue, it takes a long while. There are no markets for vaccines. Nobody has thought it necessary to develop a vaccine, not knowing when an epidemic will occur and how much money they will make from selling a few hundred vaccines.

This construct that has been developed is taken from the previous outbreaks' strains. Nobody has done a pre vaccine trial in animals in the current outbreak in Liberia and Sierra Leone. The pre-vaccine trial in animals that have been done was from strains from previous outbreaks, but since the strain in the current outbreak is 97% similar to the previous ones, we can go ahead. The protein that has been selected is 97% similar to all previous outbreaks.

Will the constructs be protective against the current or future strain?

The construct is much more prevalent than the current strain therefore it is robust. The construct is engineered such that it does not replicate itself.

We show a picture of the disease to the body. The body sees it as an enemy and is ready to fight it, so next time when the real disease shows up, the body raises its defences and starts to fight it. The trials will include children but not at this early stage.

Prolonged bleeding in some participants

The white blood cells are being boosted by the vaccine but some smaller cells had a reduction in numbers. It was at the lower level of normal and went back up within a week.

Will the trial meet international standards?

The longest time you can have a certificate without renewing it is three years and we all have our certificates. Besides protocols are being followed and being monitored by the FDA and the GHS Ethics Committee.

DR AMMA EDWIN, *Ghana Health Service Ethics Review Committee*

Our mandate is to protect study participants. Prospective research participants are given information so that they can give informed consent. Researchers are required to give an Information sheet which must state the duration, who to contact, withdrawal from the study among other information. The sheet also explains the risks and benefits and the compensations to be given.

BENEFITS

Those who have not been vaccinated against Hepatitis B will get free Hepatitis B vaccines.

The GHC 200.00 is given so that it is not too little nor too much. The GHC 200.00 is for a scheduled visit. In between visits if a participant calls at a study centre for anything he/she is given GHC30.00. There is a comprehensive insurance package. Anytime you visit a hospital for any sickness you do not pay out of pocket. You can withdraw at any time. Nobody will be forced to take part in this trial.

DELESE MIMI DARKO, *Acting Director, Food and Drugs Authority*

Our mandate under the Public Health Act, (Act 815) 2012 sections 150 to 160 includes the approval of vaccine trials. We have done a whole lot of trials since 2003. We are now looking to do trials in hypertension. We examine your proposal which is also called protocol. We look at Phase 1, 2, 3, and approve. Even after licensing we monitor Phase 4 to examine the safety of the medicine on the market. Presently Paracetamol is one of the most dangerous drugs on the market.

Ghana, Kenya, Uganda, and Tanzania all met for the Phase 1 forum. We came together with the sponsors and the sponsors answered the questions.

The research centres also came from all the participating countries to answer questions. The phase 1 process involved USFDA, Health Canada, the European Medical Agency and other similar organisations. We did that because we did not want Kenya for example to raise some issue with their study centre which we also had in our query list but we may not be there to hear it and get answers. We give approval normally for 18 months. They have seven months to start and complete recruitment. If they could not start and needed an extension of time they will tell us the reasons but in this case we all know why they have not started. If an incidence occurs with one of the participants and you do not report it after three months the FDA will sanction you.

The FDA has been designated as a Regional Centre of Research Excellence in the whole of Africa together with Zimbabwe.

QUESTIONS AND ANSWERS

Question: JOHN TSRAKASU, *Scientist*

I will term what we are doing here as damage control. When things like this happen then people come on air and say things. People went on air and said things more defensive than scientific. You should employ a public relations team for your job. Those professionals among us who are in politics should make sure our political coats are removed when we are talking about professional issues.

We saw a lot of agitations from Parliament and we were not pleased at all. How do you manage to get high profile people to receive the vaccines as an example.

Question: DJAN PHILIP, *Student, University of Health and Allied Sciences, (UHAS)*

What will be the duration before the third stage is concluded and a vaccine licensed.

Question: EDWIN OPEKU, *Ho*

Before the applicant comes out officially the FDA must give an endorsement. How did the news come into the public domain before the endorsement?

Question: JOHNSON AYAYI, *Ho*

What arrangements do you have to give disabled persons, especially hearing impaired people the information about the process?

Answer: DR AMMA EDWIN *Ghana Health Service Ethics Review Committee*

The information out there that people contacted Prof Binka and he gave information about the trial is not true. If a scientist wants that data and they use it themselves then they will be in a conflict of interest situation. What Rawlings got was not an experimented vaccine, it was an approved vaccine.

Answer: DR ABRAHAM HODGESON, *Director of Research, GHS*

The journalists got the information out before the process was completed.

Answer: PROF BINKA, *Vice Chancellor, University of Health and Allied Sciences (UHAS)*

I wish those who were supposed to have received the vaccine will be here to show us their mobile phones? The pre-clinical trial in animals was in 16 chimpanzees and they were all safe. Some doctors have written to me saying "give us the experimental vaccine outside the trial process because we are the ones at risk, not the general public. How can you give it to midwives alone or cocoa farmers alone? Are they representatives of the general population?"

Answer: PROF KWADWO KORAM, *Noguchi Memorial Institute for Medical Research, Legon*

Some of us have argued that vaccine trials are too heavily regulated. The state in which we are now, we do not use populations in the group of disabled persons for vaccine trials. The results in chimpanzees were so good so we are now trying to study the candidate vaccine in the human population.

Question: JAMES AMEWUDA, *Ho*

Is it possible to take away the GHC 200.00 and mobile phone? I do not want the compensation package. Do I qualify?

Question: SAM KUSH, *Shine FM 96.9, Akatsi*

How can you differentiate a fever caused by a trial vaccine from a fever caused by a disease?

Where are we setting these people from to come for these public education fora?

After the vaccines were given to the chimpanzees how did they develop the immunity?

Will you go back to Hohoe and Kintampo?

PROF BINKA, *Vice Chancellor, University of Health and Allied Sciences (UHAS)*

Universities undertake research; we are not a secondary school. Prof Binka said this in answer to why the trial is being held in Hohoe.

Answer: DR AMMA EDWIN, *Ghana Health Service Ethics Review Committee*

Even if you do not want the money, you still have to take it.

Answer: PROF KWADWO KORAM, *Noguchi Memorial Institute for Medical Research, Legon*

The disease is going down even in the affected countries but we want to be sure that this vaccine gives you certain protections.

Answer: PROF BINKA, *Vice Chancellor, University of Health and Allied Sciences (UHAS)*

If you have any form, please call any of us and we will come and educate you on the issues.

DR NUETEY, CHAIRMAN'S CLOSING REMARKS

The Hohoe site has been approved to carry out the Ebola trial. There is news in the foreign press that Ghanaians are kicking against the Ebola trial. I believe that we shall go from here to spread the good news of the Ebola vaccine trial.

After this last answer Ms Afua Djansi Asamoah said the closing prayer at exactly 1:00PM.

ANALYSIS AND IMPRESSION

Our analysis and impression on the proposed Ebola Vaccine Trial and its aftermath will focus on the following areas;

1. legal and regulatory framework
2. transparency
3. public education

These were the areas of contention as far as the public was concerned and they are indeed interconnected.

The confusion/wahala was largely self-inflicted.

The general public is not aware of the regulatory protocols. They do not know the steps involved nor the remit or identity of the various agencies.

Furthermore, the public is suspicious of its public officers and agencies on account of our national history.

The situation is not helped either by the conspiracy theories and understandable panic surrounding the Ebola epidemic.

There is also the perception that there is not enough distance between researchers, sponsors and regulators. The perception is that as public officers, they have a cosy relationship and the interests of the public are largely secondary.

For example, the perception is that the same researchers, regulators and sponsors at different times wear different hats. In Kintampo, we were told that Ghanaian scientists had assisted the sponsor in choosing trial participants for GSK.

In addition, the public is not sure when individual professionals are acting as academics, or employees of the GHS or MOH or as private consultants.

Therefore, even when the paperwork is produced to support regulatory protocols, it may be helpful if the composition of decision making committees is evident.

This will enhance transparency. Transparency also occurs when researchers disclose their interests when they author an academic paper for publication.

Pursuant to the above is again transparency with respect to financial rewards for investigators and participants in trial.

We have been told that a bid was won to conduct the trial but we have not been told who won the bid. Was it an individual, the research centre, the GHS, the MOH or a university?

What was the quantum of the bid?

How is it to be apportioned bearing in mind that state institutions and state personnel are involved in the trial.

The question of how much participants will be paid and why that is different from the amounts paid in the US and Europe will never go away.

Is this not an international trial that will benefit everybody?

We already have the anticipated benefits to Ghana- educational and economic.

Clarity on the above matters has not been evident from the forums held to date.

The public relations and public education aspect of the trial prior to the forums has been a disaster.

There is enough blame to go around. The situation was precipitated by professionals who gave short shrift to genuine questions raised by a concerned lay populace.

The initial mistakes made by the professionals in their responses led to an adversarial situation that has not been easy to change even though a lot of progress has been made through the forums.

The international image of our country as a destination for scientific research took a further dent when a significant number of our political leaders made ill-advised public comments to express their genuine concern.

This added fuel to the fire.

Again the public forums have assisted in recalibrating this unfortunate state of affairs.

The media has been unsatisfactory and perfunctory in its reportage since the story broke. Indeed, even at the public forums their performance was consistently sub-standard.

This has led to inaccurate information that has worsened an already difficult situation. It raises the fundamental question as to their calibre and the quality of their training.

It is obvious that since we are a developing country, there is an urgent need to build our national capacity in science reporting. The serious nature of the responsibility that falls on journalists should engender us to limit the study of journalism to second degree holders.

A poorly prepared person with a pen or microphone or camera is not harmless and we should always remember that.

The take home lesson is that our professionals, journalists and politicians need to have didactic information on issues and a thorough and well grounded understanding of the concrete nature of our society before embarking on projects or commenting or reporting on them to the public.

They ought to consider the interests of the public as supreme and be circumspect and accurate at all times.

CONCLUSION

One thing that was missing is the presentation of documentary evidence to back all the claims made by the government representatives. For example, when the Ghana Health Service Ethics Review Committee speaks about granting ethical approvals, they should next time back it up with a sample approval letter or real approval letter that was issued some time ago. Ditto for the Food and Drugs Authority (FDA). The FDA spoke authoritatively about formal steps they had taken and documents issued but none was shown to the audience. If there had been a PowerPoint presentation of such a document, or even if photocopies had been issued to the media and the audience during the forums, it would have helped discerning members of the general public ascertain the truth. Given the context that there is little to no obligation on civil/public servants to release official documents, the media may continue to speculate and spread misinformation.

AUTHORS' PROFILE

Isaac Ato Mensah is an independent scholar and journalist.

Ahmed Naeem Abdul-Ghafaar is an author, Emergency Medical Technician, journalist and law student.

Ekow Arthur-Aidoo is a journalist, lawyer and blogger.

Emmanuel Amoh-Kwaning is a web designer and communication design expert working with writersghana.com.

Stella Owusu Kwarteng is a public relations/marketing professional working with Fidelity Bank in Ghana.

www.ingramcontent.com/pod-product-compliance
Lightning Source LLC
Chambersburg PA
CBHW071950210526
45479CB00003B/883
* 9 7 9 8 3 3 3 5 3 6 8 0 8 *